TONSILLECTOMY RECOVERY NUTRITION

A Comprehensive Guide On Navigating Healing Strategies And Nutritional Support For Ear And Throat Health

DR LUCAS KAYCE

DISCLAIMER

This book about illness and nutrition is not meant to replace expert medical advice, diagnosis, or treatment; rather, it is meant purely for informational reasons. This book's content is founded on broad concepts and recommendations for managing diseases and nutrition.

Before adopting any major dietary or lifestyle changes, readers are recommended to speak with a qualified healthcare provider, such as a licensed physician or registered dietitian, especially if they have pre-existing medical concerns. Everybody has different health demands, so what works for one person might not work for another.

The use of the information provided in this book may have unfavorable repercussions or consequences, for which the author and publisher disclaim all liability. No disease is meant to be identified, treated, cured, or prevented by the information provided.

The book may include contain references to medical literature or research findings; however readers are urged to independently confirm this material and contact reliable sources.

It is important to remember that the fields of nutrition and medicine are always changing, and that new findings could have an impact on the advice offered in this book. As a result, readers are urged to keep up with the most recent advancements in healthcare and, when in doubt, seek professional counsel.

By reading this book, readers agree that they are in charge of their own health decisions and release the author and publisher from any liability arising from the use of the material in the book, whether direct or indirect.

TABLE OF CONTENTS

ABOUT THE BOOK

A crucial component of post-surgical care is covered in the book Tonsillectomy Recovery Nutrition, which highlights the role that a healthy diet plays in the healing process. Setting the scene, the Introduction describes the goal of the book as assisting readers in navigating the complexities of post-tonsillectomy recuperation with an emphasis on dietary issues.

A thorough explanation of the tonsillectomy process, the causes of its frequent occurrence and a thorough recuperation schedule are given. Readers must grasp this background information to fully understand the upcoming, which explore the nutritional components of rehabilitation.

The role of nutrition in the healing process is discussed. Particular nutrients that are essential for the recovery from a tonsillectomy are identified, such as proteins, vitamins A, C, and D, minerals iron and zinc, and adequate hydration.

For those who wish to maximize their dietary intake while recovering, this chapter is an essential resource.

The book covers the practical aspects of getting ready for recovery after a tonsillectomy, including meal planning ahead of time, stockpiling nutrient-rich foods, and preoperative nutrition. By taking the initiative, people may make sure they are ready to assist their bodies while they recuperate.

Focuses on immediate post-operative nutrition, including the value of hydration, a clear liquid diet, and the gradual switch to soft foods. These insights help readers make decisions that are well-informed during the crucial early stages of rehabilitation.

Using a practical approach, the book offers meal ideas and recipes for soft diets. This helpful guide provides a range of options to help make the healing process more pleasurable and nourishing, from smoothies and blended soups to nutrient-dense purees.

The topic of managing discomfort and swelling through nutrition is covered. Anti-inflammatory foods are introduced, along with foods to avoid, and a discussion of the significance of supplements in the healing process. This chapter provides readers with techniques to lessen typical post-operative difficulties.

The book offers nutrition suggestions for the long term, looking beyond short-term healing. It offers advice on how to keep a balanced diet, check nutrient consumption, and gradually go back to a regular diet to preserve long-term well-being.

Special concerns, including adult and pediatric tonsillectomy recovery nutrition and advice on handling possible problems, are covered. These insights ensure a customized approach to rehabilitation by catering to a wide range of reader needs.

The book provides lifestyle advice for recovering from a tonsillectomy, including stress reduction, sleep, rest, and light exercise. Throughout the healing process, these all-encompassing suggestions support general well-being.

All things considered, this book is a thorough and invaluable resource that provides a methodical and knowledgeable approach to a tonsillectomy recuperation diet. It gives people the tools they need to make educated decisions and maximize their nutritional intake for a more seamless recovery process by fusing medical knowledge with useful guidance.

COMPREHENDING TONSILLECTOMY

After a tonsillectomy—a surgical operation in which the tonsils are removed—nutrition is crucial to the healing process. It is crucial to maintain a healthy diet throughout this recuperation phase because it has a direct effect on the body's capacity to mend and rebuild strength. For those undergoing tonsillectomy, a diet high in nutrients and well-balanced will help minimize complications, lessen discomfort, and speed up the healing process in general.

It is crucial to first realize the nature of the tonsillectomy process to appreciate the importance of nutrition in tonsillectomy recovery. The tiny, oval-shaped masses of tissue called tonsils are situated in the back of the throat. By capturing bacteria and viruses, they help the immune system function. A tonsillectomy is the surgical removal of these tonsils, usually as a result of ongoing infections, breathing problems, or other medical conditions. Although tonsillectomy is most usually performed on children, in certain medical circumstances, adults may also have the surgery.

SYNOPSIS OF THE TONSILLECTOMY PROCESS

A summary of the tonsillectomy process shows that the tonsils are normally removed through the mouth by the surgeon without the need for any external incisions. The treatment is usually performed under a general anesthetic. Even though tonsillectomy is thought of as a normal procedure, there is a recovery period thereafter, and patients are urged to adhere to specific instructions to promote the best possible healing.

TYPICAL CAUSES OF TONSILLECTOMY

A tonsillectomy may be performed for a variety of causes, such as recurrent tonsillitis, severe or persistent infections, breathing difficulties brought on by larger tonsils, tumors, or other abnormalities. When recommending a tonsillectomy, medical professionals carefully consider the risks and benefits and base their decision mostly on the severity and frequency of symptoms.

TIMELINE FOR RECUPERATION

Patients and their caregivers must be aware of the recovery period following a tonsillectomy. Swallowing difficulties, pain in the throat, and discomfort are possible in the early postoperative days after the surgery, although these side effects eventually go away. To avoid irritating the surgery site, a restricted diet consisting of soft and easily digestible meals is usually necessary during the first week. Patients can progressively resume a more regular diet as the days go by, making sure to stay well-hydrated and steering clear of any items that might make them uncomfortable.

It is clear how important diet is in this situation. A diet high in protein, vitamins, and minerals is necessary to help the body recover itself. Maintaining proper hydration is especially crucial to avoid dehydration, which can worsen pain and postpone healing. Yogurt, soups, and pureed fruits are examples of soft, readily chewable foods that can help satisfy nutritional needs while easing the healing process of the throat.

A healthy diet is essential for a full recovery following a tonsillectomy. Comprehending the process, the typical causes and the recuperation schedule offers a thorough understanding of the difficulties people have throughout this time. A diet high in nutrients and well-balanced not only aids in the healing process but also makes recuperation easier and more comfortable. Healthcare providers frequently offer individualized food advice, highlighting the vital connection between good nutrition and a speedy recovery following a tonsillectomy.

CHAPTER ONE

NUTRITIONAL REQUIREMENTS FOR HEALING

NUTRITION'S SIGNIFICANCE IN HEALING

Adequate nutritional intake is necessary to assist recovery following a variety of medical procedures, including surgeries like a tonsillectomy and plays a critical part in the healing process. It is impossible to overestimate the role that diet plays in healing because it directly affects the body's capacity to mend wounds, fight illness, and rebuild strength. The body's nutritional requirements frequently rise during the healing process, so it's critical to concentrate on eating a well-balanced diet that offers the nutrients required for the best possible healing.

COMPLETE PROTEIN

Protein is a crucial element in the diet that supports recuperation. Protein is essential for both the creation of new cells and tissue healing. The removal of the tonsils during a surgical operation called a tonsillectomy increases the body's requirement for protein. Consuming enough protein aids in the production of collagen, which is necessary for the healing of wounds. To encourage the best healing throughout the healing phase, foods high in lean protein, such as fish, poultry, eggs, dairy products, and lentils, should be given priority.

VITAMINS

Vitamins play an important function in healing in addition to protein. Vitamins, like vitamin C, are essential for the body's immune system and for the synthesis of collagen.

Vitamin A is necessary for tissue healing and promotes mucous membrane regeneration, both of which are impacted by tonsillectomy frequently. A varied spectrum of vitamins is ensured by including a range of fruits and vegetables in the diet, which supports general health and facilitates healing.

MINERALS

Minerals are also essential for the healing process following a tonsillectomy. A sufficient intake of calcium and phosphorus is especially crucial during the healing period to assist in the regeneration of bone tissues. These nutrients are fundamental for the health of bones. Zinc also helps to promote wound healing and the immune system. To satisfy these particular dietary requirements, foods high in minerals, such as dairy products, leafy green vegetables, nuts, and seeds, should be a part of the diet.

HYDRATION AND FLUIDS

Another crucial component of nutritional support during recovery is staying well hydrated. Drinking enough fluids is essential to avoiding dehydration, which can impede the healing process. Water is necessary for many biological processes, such as the transportation of nutrients, regulation of body temperature, and excretion of waste.

To maintain proper hydration during the post-tonsillectomy phase, people should drink lots of water in addition to other hydrating liquids such as herbal teas and broths.

Proper nutrition during tonsillectomy recuperation is critical to a speedy and complete healing process. The body's capacity to heal and rebuild strength is supported by protein, vitamins, minerals, and enough hydration. To guarantee that the body gets the nutrients it needs to promote maximum healing and reduce difficulties during the healing process, a well-balanced diet that includes a range of nutrient-dense foods is crucial.

CHAPTER TWO

GETTING READY FOR TONSILLECTOMY RECUPERATION

BEFORE SURGERY, EAT

One important part of getting ready for tonsillectomy recovery is preoperative nutrition. It is crucial to concentrate on keeping up a healthy, well-balanced diet before having the surgery. Sufficient nourishment is essential for improving the body's capacity to mend and recuperate following surgery. Speaking with a nutritionist or healthcare provider can assist create a preoperative food plan that suits each person's requirements and guarantees the body gets the nutrients it needs for the impending treatment.

PURCHASING NUTRIENT-RICH FOODS IN BULK

Purchasing a large supply of foods high in nutrients is a crucial component of the preparatory work. Increasing your supply of meals high in vitamins, minerals, and other vital nutrients will help speed up your healing.

Fruits, vegetables, whole grains, dairy products, and lean proteins are examples of these foods. These nutrient-dense foods can help the body heal more quickly by boosting tissue repair, immune system support, and energy production. Keeping your refrigerator and pantry well-stocked can guarantee that you have easy access to wholesome meals when your energy may be lower in the early stages of recuperation.

Meal planning before surgery is a doable strategy to ensure a seamless transition into the convalescence stage. Meal planning and preparation ahead of time can reduce stress and the amount of cooking that needs to be done after surgery.

To ease any pain felt when swallowing, think about concentrating on soft, easily digested foods. Smoothies, pureed foods, broths, and soups are all great ways to get those vital nutrients without overwhelming the body's healing capacity. To avoid dehydration, it's also critical to stay hydrated. Drink plenty of water, herbal teas, and electrolyte-rich beverages.

Optimizing nutritional intake during preoperative nutrition requires incorporating a variety of food types into the diet. Carbs give you energy, proteins help repair damaged tissue, and vitamins and minerals are good for your general health. Maintaining a healthy balance between macronutrient and micronutrient consumption can help the body become more resilient and prepared for the impending surgery. Processed and sugar-filled foods should be avoided in excess since they might impede the healing process and cause inflammation.

Potential dietary advice or limits from the medical team should also be taken into account. It could be recommended to some people to abstain from specific foods or drinks in the hours preceding surgery. Following these recommendations is crucial for a tonsillectomy to be both safe and effective. Furthermore, talking with the healthcare practitioner about any current dietary restrictions or worries can assist in customizing the preoperative food plan to fit individual requirements and guarantee a smooth recovery process.

A holistic strategy to improve the healing process must include preoperative nutrition, stocking up on nutrient-rich foods, and careful meal planning before tonsillectomy. A healthy diet can help patients support their body's healing processes, reduce the risk of problems, and facilitate a more seamless recovery from surgery.

CHAPTER THREE

RIGHT AFTER SURGERY NUTRITION

THE CLEAR LIQUID DIET

The recovery process greatly benefits from early post-operative nutrition, with special emphasis placed on the Clear Liquid Diet, the value of staying hydrated, and the shift to soft foods. All of these elements work together to improve the patient's general health and facilitate a speedy recovery following surgery.

The post-operative dietary strategy generally starts with the Clear Liquid Diet. The main items on this diet are liquid-based, readily digested foods including gelatin, clear liquids, and broths. Its goal is to minimize digestive system stress while supplying vital fluids.

This stage permits the gastrointestinal tract to gradually return to normal function following surgery helps guard against dehydration and ensures appropriate hydration. A clear liquid diet also facilitates the progressive reintroduction of more substantial foods after the period of fasting before surgery.

THE VALUE OF HYDRATION

An essential component of initial post-operative care is hydration. Maintaining physiological processes, promoting wound healing, and avoiding problems like dehydration all depend on adequate fluid intake. To replace lost fluids and electrolytes, intravenous fluids are frequently given during and right after surgery. Encourage the patient to drink small sips of water and other clear liquids once they can handle oral intake. Staying hydrated promotes a more seamless recovery by supporting the body's general metabolic functions and helps the body flush out any leftover anesthetic effects.

MAKING THE SWITCH TO SOFT FOODS

The clear liquid phase is followed by a gradual transition to soft meals based on the patient's tolerance of increasingly complex nutrients. Soft foods are less taxing on the digestive tract and can help avert issues like nausea and vomiting following surgery. Mashed potatoes, pureed veggies, yogurt, and soft fruits are a few examples of foods that are considered soft. During this stage of the post-operative nutrition plan, items that could be difficult to digest can be avoided while the gastrointestinal tract can adjust to a more diversified diet. It's critical to keep an eye on how the patient responds to soft meals and modify the diet to each person's tolerance and level of recovery.

The initial post-operative nutrition regimen, which includes the Clear Liquid Diet, a focus on hydration, and a gradual switch to soft foods, is a meticulously thought-out and supervised procedure. Together, these elements facilitate the best possible recovery following surgery, guard against problems, and strengthen the body's natural healing processes.

CHAPTER FOUR

RECIPES AND MENU IDEAS FOR A SOFT DIET

DRINKS & CONCOCTIONS

Smoothies and blended soups are great choices for people following a low-fat diet. These adaptable, simple-to-prepare foods offer a straightforward method to add a range of nutrients without sacrificing texture. Smoothies are a tasty and refreshing alternative. They are usually produced by combining fruits, vegetables, yogurt, or milk. They can be altered to suit dietary requirements and personal tastes. Protein powder, bananas, berries, spinach, and other ingredients can be combined to create a smooth, creamy mixture that is filling and healthy.

Conversely, for individuals looking for a savory substitute, blended soups offer a cozy and warm option. Soups that are smooth and simple to digest can be made by cooking and pureeing vegetables, lentils, and proteins. Not only do herbs and spices improve flavor, but they also add nutrients to the dish. Prominent choices include velvety tomato soup, butternut squash soup, or a substantial lentil soup, all of which can be customized to meet particular dietary needs.

GELATIN AND PUDDINGS

Desserts like puddings and gelatin are delicious sweets that those following a soft diet can enjoy. These choices have a pleasant texture and are simple to prepare, making them ideal for people who have trouble swallowing or chewing. Puddings can be flavored with vanilla, chocolate, or fruit puree and created using several bases, including rice, almond, or milk. To enhance texture and nutritional value, try adding foods like chia seeds.

Desserts made with gelatin, sometimes called "jello," are another delightfully soft choice. Collagen is the source of the protein known as gelatin, which, when combined with liquid and refrigerated, solidifies into a soft, palatable pudding. It comes in a variety of flavors, and for extra flavor and nutrition, you may top it with yogurt or bits of fruit. These desserts are a good option for people who have trouble swallowing solid foods because they not only offer a sweet delight but also help with hydration.

RICH IN NUTRIENT PUREES

Because they provide a concentrated dose of vital vitamins and minerals, nutrient-dense purees are essential to soft diets. Foods are made into purees by mixing them until they have a smooth consistency that facilitates digestion. Nutrient-dense purees made from vegetables, fruits, lean meats, and grains can be made to meet specific nutritional requirements.

Sweet potatoes, carrots, and peas are good choices for vegetable purees since they can be boiled and blended to make a colorful and tasty side dish. Fruit purees, like mashed bananas or applesauce, offer natural sugars and fiber in addition to sweetness. Proteins can be pureed by blending cooked meats, fish, or lentils, which provides a soft, high-protein option for people following certain dietary guidelines.

There are many different and fun soft diet recipes and meal ideas that include anything from puddings, gelatin sweets, and nutrient-dense purees to smoothies and blended soups. These options ensure a varied and nutrient-dense diet, which promotes overall well-being in addition to meeting the needs of people with particular dietary restrictions.

CHAPTER FIVE

USING NUTRITION TO MANAGE PAIN AND SWELLING

ANTI-INFLAMMATORY FOODS

Using nutrition to reduce pain and swelling requires a planned strategy that includes anti-inflammatory foods, avoiding particular trigger foods, and using supplements to speed up healing.

The daily diet's use of anti-inflammatory items is a crucial component of this dietary approach. These meals are essential for reducing inflammation and enhancing general health. Berries, especially blueberries and cherries, are considered high-antioxidant and anti-inflammatory fruits.

 In a similar vein, omega-3 fatty acids, which have been demonstrated to lessen inflammation in the body, are widely present in fatty fish like sardines, mackerel, and salmon. Because leafy greens like spinach and kale are high in vitamins and minerals, eating them can also help promote an anti-inflammatory diet.

ITEMS TO STEER CLEAR OF

On the other hand, knowing which foods to avoid and how they can worsen inflammation is just as crucial to controlling pain and swelling. Processed foods that are heavy in refined carbohydrates, trans fats, and sodium can aggravate inflammation. It is important to limit consumption of these things in addition to avoiding refined carbs and saturated fats. Furthermore, because some nightshade vegetables, like tomatoes and peppers, contain substances that might aggravate inflammation, some may find it helpful to reduce their intake of these vegetables.

SUPPLEMENTS FOR RECUPERATION

When it comes to reducing pain and swelling, supplements can help. Omega-3 fatty acid supplements are well-known for their anti-inflammatory qualities and can be especially helpful in aiding in recuperation. They are made from algae or fish oil. The curcumin-containing spice turmeric is another substance that has demonstrated potential for lowering inflammation. Notable supplements for those who want to control pain and swelling with food include vitamin D, which regulates the immune system, and ginger, which has anti-inflammatory and antioxidant qualities.

A thorough nutritional strategy for controlling pain and swelling entails choosing anti-inflammatory meals carefully, avoiding pro-inflammatory foods, and incorporating recovery-promoting vitamins. People can take proactive measures to manage inflammation-related problems and promote general well-being by giving priority to these dietary components.

CHAPTER SIX

LONG-TERM DIETARY APPROACHES

RETURNING GRADUALLY TO A REGULAR DIET

A gradual return to a regular diet following a period of restricted or specialized nutrition is essential to ensure a seamless transition and avoid any negative effects on the body. Differing eating habits suddenly can cause digestive distress and metabolic difficulties. Reintroducing a wider variety of foods gradually reduces the chance of gastrointestinal distress and gives the digestive system time to adjust. This strategy is especially pertinent to people who have followed certain diets for weight control or medical purposes.

The methodical reintroduction of food groups, beginning with readily digestible and well-tolerated options, is part of the gradual return to a regular diet. For example, patients recovering from surgery or certain medical problems might start with bland, readily digestible foods and work their way up to more varied, nutrient-dense options. In addition to assisting in the identification of any potential sensitivities or intolerances that may have arisen during the restricted period, this staged approach supports the body's ability to digest various nutrients.

SUSTAINING AN EQUILIBRIUM DIET

Eating a balanced diet is essential for good health and well-being in general. Consuming a range of nutrients in the right amounts, such as carbs, proteins, fats, vitamins, and minerals, is part of a balanced diet. Maintaining this equilibrium guarantees that the body gets the components it needs for maximum performance, from generating energy to bolstering the immune system. Another important function of a well-rounded diet is to prevent nutritional deficits and related health problems.

Dietary balance is achieved by including a variety of foods from each of the major food groups. Whole grains, lean meats, fruits, veggies, and healthy fats are examples of this. Aside from preventing overindulgence, controlling portion sizes is also crucial because eating too much of even healthful meals can cause imbalances and unintended weight gain. Additionally, by encouraging a positive relationship with food, mindful eating techniques like observing fullness and hunger cues support a balanced diet.

TRACKING THE INTAKE OF NUTRIENTS

A crucial element of any successful long-term nutrition plan is keeping an eye on nutrient consumption. It entails being aware of the kinds and amounts of nutrients that are regularly ingested. With this knowledge, people can make educated decisions about their diets, guaranteeing that they get the nutrients they need while avoiding excesses or shortages. It becomes more important to monitor nutrient intake for those who have certain medical issues, follow certain diets, or have performance objectives.

Nutrient consumption can be tracked using a variety of instruments and techniques, from contemporary smartphone apps to conventional food journals. With the use of these tools, people may keep track of their meals, evaluate the nutritional value of various foods, and pinpoint areas that could require improvements. Furthermore, consulting certified dietitians or other medical specialists can offer tailored advice on dietary requirements based on lifestyle choices, personal health objectives, and any underlying medical issues. A long-term, sustainable, and health-promoting approach to nutrition is ensured by routine evaluation and dietary adjustment.

CHAPTER SEVEN

PARTICULAR POINTS TO REMEMBER

NUTRITION FOR PEDIATRIC TONSILLECTOMY RECOVERY

A pediatric tonsillectomy is a frequent surgical surgery used to treat conditions like breathing difficulties during sleep or recurrent throat infections. Children recovering from tonsillectomy must pay close attention to their diet. It's critical to concentrate on a healthy, readily digested food after the treatment. It is advised to eat soft, cold, and non-irritating foods to reduce pain and accelerate healing.

Encourage your child to drink lots of fluids, such as water and clear broths, to stay hydrated. Eat foods that are cold and soft, such as yogurt, popsicles, and ice cream, to soothe sore throats and make sure you're getting enough calories. Foods that are hot, spicy, or acidic should be avoided since they may aggravate the surgical site that is healing.

Smoothies, mashed veggies, and pureed fruits are nutrient-rich foods that can help meet the child's total nutritional requirements as they heal. Maintaining a well-rounded diet that prioritizes vitamins and minerals boosts immunity and expedites healing. Additionally, caregivers should keep an eye on the child's eating patterns and change them as necessary to suit their comfort level and preferences.

ADULT RECUPERATED TONSILLECTOMY DIET

Recovery nutrition is equally important for an adult tonsillectomy to guarantee a speedy healing process. Compared to children, adults may feel more discomfort and require longer recovery periods. Soft and readily chewable foods are recommended during the early stages of recovery. Maintaining sufficient nutrition becomes vital for individuals having tonsillectomy, as it aids in tissue repair, lowers the risk of problems, and increases overall well-being. This covers foods like pasta, mashed potatoes, and soups. Staying well hydrated is crucial to avoiding dehydration, particularly in the early postoperative phase when swallowing could be difficult. Foods that are abrasive or rough are not recommended as they may aggravate the surgical site.

Foods high in protein, such as dairy, eggs, and lean meats, are essential for healing because they promote tissue repair. The best healing is facilitated by eating a diet that is well-balanced and rich in different vitamins and minerals. While eating a healthy diet is important, people should also pay attention to their bodies' needs and modify their eating patterns to suit their comfort levels.

HANDLING DIFFICULTIES

Even with the best of intentions, problems can occur in both adult and pediatric tonsillectomy patients after their procedure. People and others who are caring for them must be aware of such problems and seek immediate medical assistance when necessary.

Bleeding is a typical problem that can happen in the initial days following surgery. It is critical to get in touch with a healthcare professional right once if there is significant bleeding. In these situations, staying hydrated is even more important to avoid the consequences of blood loss.

Another worry is infections, for which people should watch out for symptoms like fever, increasing pain, or ongoing sore throats. Infections caused by bacteria may be treated with antibiotics, and close observation is necessary to stop the infection from spreading.

Complications may also arise from dehydration, particularly in those who have difficulty consuming fluids. It is essential to have open lines of contact with medical professionals to discuss any concerns and get advice on how to handle difficulties. To guarantee the best possible result, further medical procedures or changes to the rehabilitation plan can be required in specific cases.

CHAPTER EIGHT

LIVING SUGGESTIONS FOR TONSILLECTOMY RECUPERATION

SLEEP AND REST

A tonsillectomy is a surgical surgery in which the tonsils are removed. A successful recovery from this procedure depends on getting enough sleep and rest. It's crucial to get lots of rest after surgery so that the body can recuperate properly. Getting enough sleep promotes tissue regeneration and lessens any potential discomfort during the process. It is suggested that patients follow the rest period prescribed by their healthcare experts, which usually consists of a few days of lowered activity.

Due to the effects of anesthetic and the body's natural reaction to the surgical procedure, people may feel tired and drowsy in the early days of their tonsillectomy recovery. Establishing a cozy and supportive sleeping space is essential, and using additional pillows to keep the head raised may help reduce sore throats.

Furthermore, maintaining hydration is essential since it can help ward off dehydration, a common surgical side effect, and promote general health during the convalescence phase.

MODERATE EXERCISE

Although recuperation following a tonsillectomy must prioritize rest, mild exercise can also be helpful. Short walks and other light exercise can enhance circulation, reduce stiffness, and promote general wellbeing. But it's important to stay away from hard workouts and other activities that could aggravate the throat or hinder the healing process.

In addition to promoting a quicker recovery by preventing muscle atrophy, mild physical activity also helps to prevent complications like blood clots.

Before beginning any physical activity, it is imperative to speak with medical professionals to make sure that it is in line with the patient's recovery plan and advice.

STRESS MANAGEMENT

Since stress can impede the healing process, stress management is important for tonsillectomy recovery. During their recuperation, patients should give priority to engaging in activities that enhance their mental and physical health. Stress reduction methods like deep breathing exercises, mindfulness, and meditation can be helpful.

It's critical to discuss any worries or anxieties you may have regarding the healing process honestly with your healthcare professionals. Positivity is enhanced by realistic expectations and knowledge of the anticipated timetable for recovery. Taking part in enjoyable and soothing activities, like reading, listening to music, or spending time with loved ones, can also help reduce stress and create an atmosphere that is favorable for healing.